commitment to medical
education.

CW00361919

Pocket Picture Guides

Forensic Medicine

Bernard Knight
MD, BCh, FRC Path, DMJ, Barrister-at-Law

Professor of Forensic Pathology
The Welsh National School of Medicine
Royal Infirmary, Cardiff, UK

Gower Medical Publishing · London · New York · 1985

© Copyright 1985 by Gower Medical Publishing Ltd.
34-42 Cleveland Street, London W1P 5FB, England.

Distribution limited to United Kingdom.

ISBN 0-906923-42-5

British Library Cataloguing in Publication Data
Knight, Bernard, 19-- –
    Forensic medicine. –
    (Pocket picture guide to clinical medicine; v.8)
    1. Medical jurisprudence
    I. Title   II. Series
    614.1   RA1051

Project Editor: Fiona Carr
     Designer: Leslie Watts
    Illustrators: Edwina Hannam
                Karen Cochrane

Printed in Italy by Imago Publishing Ltd.

Contents

Within a small volume such as this, it is obviously impossible to offer a comprehensive account of forensic medicine and pathology, which is provided elsewhere by many larger textbooks and monographs. The object of this atlas is to illustrate a representative selection of forensic medical situations and to comment briefly upon them, by means of both the captions to the photographs and by a short summary before each chapter.

A concious effort has been made to select relatively common forensic situations rather than the exotic and to avoid reference to any particular medico-legal systems, which might thereby limit the geographical appeal of the book. In addition, attention is concentrated upon **external** appearances, rather than internal pathology, again to appeal to the widest possible range of doctors.

Clinicians of all types frequently encounter medico-legal problems, even though they might not recognise them as such at the time. Apart from the daily administrative legal matters such as the certification of death, reporting to the coroner or other medico-legal agency, cremation, other types of certification etc., there is the ever-present spectre of negligence allegations. Law enforcement agencies, lawyers and others require medical reports and statements and sometimes the doctor has to give testimony in court upon his observations. All these matters can be a strain if the doctor has not gained some familiarity with various types of trauma and systematic ways of writing descriptions of that trauma, early in his or her medical career. A pictorial approach to the most common of these problems is offered in these pages.

Introduction

Forensic medicine, which embraces both pathology and clinical practice, is largely the study of trauma, whether it be assault, homicide, rape or the effects of suicide or accident. The broad category of trauma includes poisoning and the effects of heat, cold and electricity. Sudden unexpected death is also a substantial part of forensic work, but is outside the scope of this small atlas.

A doctor may be called to see either a live patient or a dead body in circumstances which may have profound medico-legal consequences. Examples are the battered child, the alleged victim of a sexual offence, the victim of a violent assault, traffic or industrial accident or a dead body which lies in a situation which may be either overtly suspicious or at least unexplained.

Unfortunately, not all doctors anticipate the possible legal sequelae and make an inadequate examination. Many cases are on record where doctors have missed severe injuries in a live or dead patient. Not only is an adequate examination necessary for the benefit of the patient - who may sue if he is dissatisfied - but in case of crime or unnatural death, the doctor may attract the censure of law enforcement authorities for his omission to carry out even the most elementary examination.

A good examination is of little use if there is no satisfactory report made by the doctor. Such a report (made after due regard to the needs of medical confidentiality) should be legible, dated and written with clarity and objectivity. If the doctor does not claim to be an expert, he should confine himself to facts and not venture into the realms of opinion or speculation.

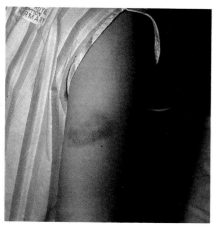

Fig. 1 An injury of a live victim – a bruise on an abused child, caused by an adult hand gripping the upper arm. This is a typical lesion in both battered children and in adult fights, the contusion being caused on the soft skin by thumb and/or finger pressure. The upper arm is a convenient 'handle' for gripping by an assailant.

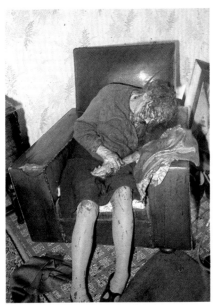

Fig. 2 The scene of a murder, where an old lady suffered gross head injuries from an iron bar in the course of a robbery. A doctor called to such a scene has the opportunity to relate the injuries to the surroundings. He is able to see the direction and extent of blood splashes on adjacent furniture and walls, to observe the posture of the body and to measure environmental temperature and other conditions, none of which would be possible if the body were first seen in the mortuary.

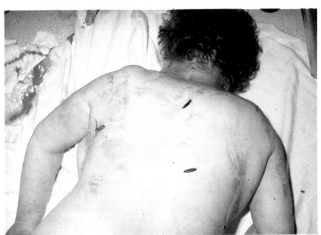

Fig. 3 A murder completely missed by the family physician, who issued a death certificate for 'epistaxis'. Doctors called to a death should at least identify the source of profuse bleeding before being satisfied that death is due to natural causes. The three stab wounds here were found by the funeral directors. The injury near the axilla is V-shaped due to twisting of the knife before removal.

Identification

Although the identity of most subjects, whether living or dead, is known from witnesses or the circumstances, there are often problems, for example when a live patient is found unconscious. More commonly, the age of either a child or an adult may be in dispute. Eligibility for pensions, for school or military service or for immigration matters may have to be resolved on medical criteria of age if no certificates or reliable documented proof is available.

In the dead, it may be necessary to identify intact, decomposed or even skeletalised corpses. Where homicide has occurred, the killer may have deliberately mutilated or disposed of the body so that putrefaction renders recognition impossible. Even in non-criminal deaths, post-mortem decomposition, especially in water, may require extensive medico-anthropological investigation.

The following facts must be determined if possible:

Sex. Except in rare cases, the genitalia indicate the sex. In decomposed bodies, the uterus is the last organ to putrefy. In skeletal material, the skull and pelvis offer more than a 90% chance of correct sexing.

Height. The stature of a person can be measured directly when intact. There may be several centimetres difference between live and dead length. In skeletons, measurement of the assembled skeleton may give an approximate height, supplemented by calculations on long bones, using anatomical formulae.

Age. This important criterion may be most accurately estimated in both the living and dead in the younger subject. In fetuses and infants, age may be estimated to within weeks by ossification centres and body size. In later childhood and youth, tooth eruption and epiphyseal fusion are the criteria, making allowance for sex, race and geography. After the third decade, accuracy declines greatly and specialist anatomical expertise is needed.

Race. Differentiation is difficult in skeletal material, apart from tooth changes in mongoloid races and facial and long bone measurements in negroids.

Personal identity. Numerous criteria exist, including scars, tattoos, deformities, fingerprints, frontal sinus patterns, hair, eyes, and of course teeth. The latter are very important, especially in mass disasters such as air crashes where mutilation and burning may obscure other signs.

IDENTIFICATION

Live person

Sex

Stature

Race

Weight

Age

Individuality   Hair, eyes, tattoos, scars,
operations, deformities, naevi

Dead body

INTACT - as for live person

DECOMPOSED

Sex   Uterus, nuclear chromatin

Age   Arthritis, arterial degeneration

SKELETAL FEATURES

?Human

Sex   Skull, pelvis, femora

Race   Teeth, skull

Height   Direct measurement
Calculation from limbs

Age   Teeth , ossification centres
Epiphyseal fusion

Individuality   Frontal sinuses
Skull radiography, teeth
Old fractures , bone disease
and deformities

Fig. 4 Diagram of the criteria for the identification of a body.
These may in part be applicable to a live person, where because of
coma, immaturity, language or refusal to co-operate, direct evidence
is unobtainable.

4

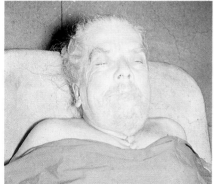

Fig. 5 Facial appearances may be deceptive in determining sex. This person was female and naturally, the physical features of the rest of the body would clarify the matter, However, deliberate or accidental mutilation, decomposition or skeletalisation may obscure the determination.

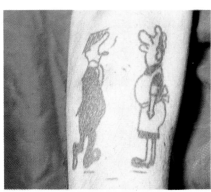

Fig. 6 Tattoos may be useful identifying factors in both living and dead. Both the general nature and the individuality may help, as in this 'Andy Capp' design. Military, religious and ethnic themes and individual names can be of considerable assistance.

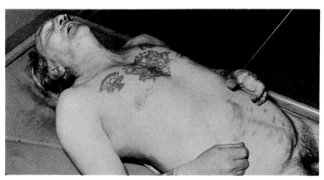

Fig. 7 Surgical scars and amputations may aid identification, as in this man who had two fingers missing and a large abdominal scar, together with many tattoos. Where identity is unknown, all possible evidence must be accumulated from every physical finding.

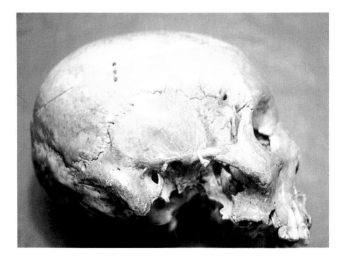

Fig. 8 A male skull showing the heavy bone structure, the rough surface for stronger muscle attachment, the heavier brow ridges, the more sloping forehead and especially the large mastoid process. Naturally, there is a wide spectrum of variation, but sexing is over 90% accurate when the skull is used.

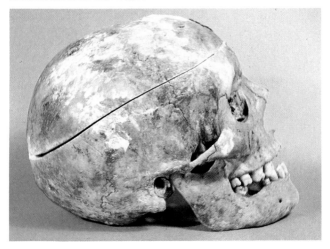

Fig. 9 A female skull, showing the smooth, rounded outline, high forehead, absent eyebrow ridges and small mastoid. Caution must be used where certain ethnic groups are involved, as the sexual differences in skeletons from the Indian sub-continent may be slight.

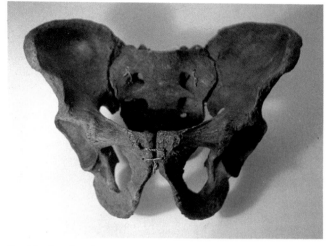

Fig. 10 A male pelvis, which is more upright than the female, with a narrower, heart-shaped inlet. The subpubic angle between the inferior rami is narrow, being less than a right-angle.

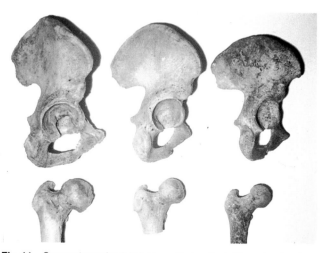

Fig. 11 Comparison of pelvic bones – that on the left is male, showing a larger, more laterally-facing acetabulum, a higher iliac blade and a narrow sciatic notch. The centre bone is a reference female example, that on the right is from a murder victim buried for many years, which reveals even more obvious female features.

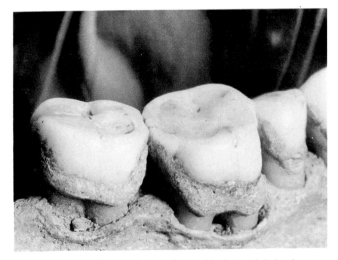

Fig. 12 Attrition of the occlusal surfaces of teeth in old skeletal remains. In Western Europe, such remains are almost always older than the mid-19th century, when a coarse diet including flour containing stone dust from milling caused severe wear of the chewing surfaces.

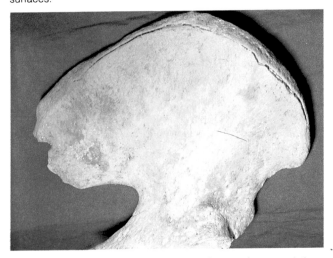

Fig. 13 Pelvic bone showing obvious male features (narrow sciatic notch) but also an indication of age. There is a line of incomplete fusion between the separately-ossified crest and blade of the ilium, suggesting an age of about 20 years.

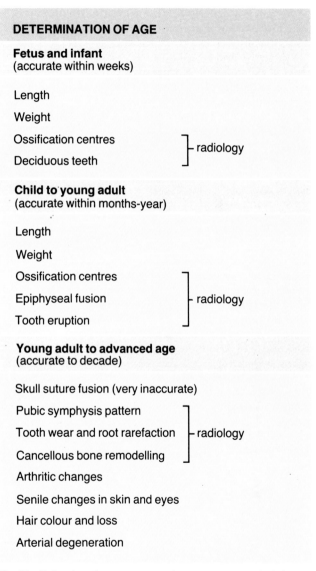

DETERMINATION OF AGE

Fetus and infant
(accurate within weeks)

Length

Weight

Ossification centres

Deciduous teeth

— radiology

Child to young adult
(accurate within months-year)

Length

Weight

Ossification centres

Epiphyseal fusion

Tooth eruption

— radiology

Young adult to advanced age
(accurate to decade)

Skull suture fusion (very inaccurate)

Pubic symphysis pattern

Tooth wear and root rarefaction

Cancellous bone remodelling

— radiology

Arthritic changes

Senile changes in skin and eyes

Hair colour and loss

Arterial degeneration

Fig. 14 Estimation of age – accuracy decreases progressively from the fetus to old age.

Post-mortem changes

Most attempts at estimating time since death rely upon post-mortem changes, though over-confidence in the accuracy of this exercise is all too common.

Hypostasis ('lividity') is the discoloration of the skin due to gravitational settling of blood in the lowest areas. It is of no use in estimating the time of death, but an abnormal colour may indicate some toxic substance.

Rigor mortis is very variable in its onset, appearing rapidly and passing off quickly in warm conditions. It usually sets in within a few hours and lasts for 2-3 days, although variation is very considerable.

Body temperature is the best criterion of time since death, though again much depends on the environmental conditions and the state of the body (clothing, posture, obesity, oedema, etc). In temperate climates, body temperature usually nears that of the surroundings by the end of the first day.

Decomposition sets in at a very variable time after death. This may be within a few hours in the tropics, but may never occur in frigid climates. In temperate conditions the 3rd-4th day usually reveals the first signs of putrefaction. Bodies in water decompose more slowly, and those buried last even longer. The usual moist putrefaction may be replaced by mummification in dry conditions and the converse may occur in water or damp places, when the adipose tissue becomes converted to 'adipocere', a soapy substance which may retain the shape of the body for many years.

Post-mortem damage must be carefully differentiated from ante-mortem wounds. In post-mortem injuries inflicted by animals, insects, moulds and physical trauma, the usual signs of bleeding and tissue reaction are absent, although differentiation may be difficult or impossible where injuries are inflicted at or immediately after death.

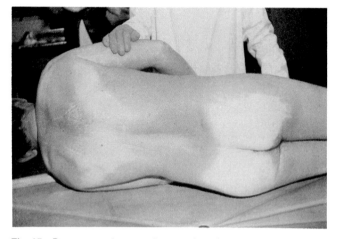

Fig. 15 Post-mortem hypostasis, sometimes incorrectly called 'lividity'. Gravitational settling of the blood after death causes the lowest areas of skin to be discoloured, except where pressure of the shoulder and buttock regions against a hard surface prevents the entry of blood into the dependent capillaries. Hypostasis may move at any time after death, if the position of the body is altered, so that the so-called 'fixation' does not necessarily occur.

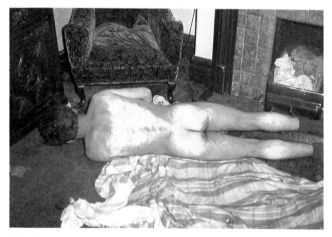

Fig. 16 Hypostasis is usually pink or purple. In cold conditions, including refrigeration after death, it may be bright red. In this photograph, it is 'cherry-red' due to carbon monoxide poisoning. Cyanide and methaemoglobinaemia also alter the colour of the hypostasis.

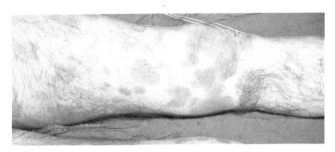

Fig. 17 Hypostasis may be blotchy on upper or lateral surfaces in the early period after death, but later coalesces and moves down to the most dependent areas. This has no significance and hypostasis is of little value in determining the time since death.

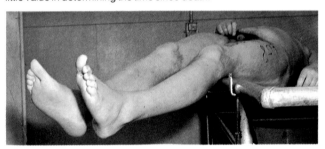

Fig. 18 Rigor mortis is a stiffening of the muscles caused by chemical changes after death, but these in turn are partly dependent upon temperature. Thus rigor is a poor index of time since death – in 'average' conditions in temperate countries, it first appears in 3-6 hours, is fully established in 12 hours, then lasts up to 2-3 days. However, great variations may occur, especially in cold conditions.

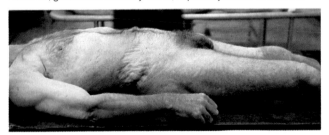

Fig. 19 The first signs of putrefaction usually appear in the right iliac fossa on the abdomen, where the caecum lies near the surface. Gut bacteria break down haemoglobin, which causes green staining. This may occur within hours in the tropics, but in colder climates may not appear for 3-4 days.

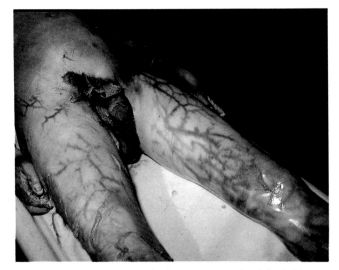

Fig. 20 More advanced putrefaction may present 'marbling' of the skin, due to putrefactive bacteria growing along the veins. This body has been recovered from water after about two weeks. Immersion markedly slows decomposition, but temperature and pollution again cause wide variation in the timing of decay.

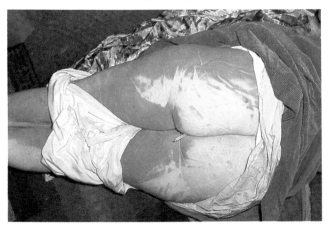

Fig. 21 Cherry-pink hypostasis in a victim of carbon monoxide poisoning. Note the chemical thermometer in the anus: the most reliable method of attempting to assess the time since death. Rectal temperature is a degree or two Centigrade higher than mouth temperature during the first few hours after death.

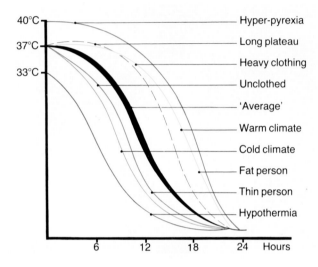

40°C	Hyper-pyrexia
37°C	Long plateau
33°C	Heavy clothing
	Unclothed
	'Average'
	Warm climate
	Cold climate
	Fat person
	Thin person
	Hypothermia

6 12 18 24 Hours

Fig. 22 Diagrammatic representation of the fall in temperature after death. The rate of fall is affected by many factors and the initial plateau may extend to up to two hours. A uniform curve only applies if the environment remains unchanged, which is rarely the case. This emphasises the risks of offering too dogmatic an opinion about the time of death.

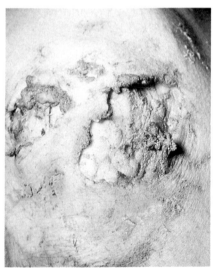

Fig. 23 Post-mortem laceration in a body recovered from the water. There is no reddening of the margins and no infiltration of blood under the edges. Naturally, any free bleeding has been washed away by the water. Such injuries are common in immersed corpses, from rough contact with underwater obstacles.

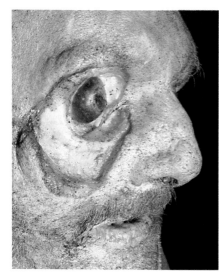

Fig. 24 Post-mortem injury caused by rats. Although initially, the police were suspicious of foul play, the absence of tissue reaction or bleeding indicates that the injury occurred after death. Close examination of the edges showed rodent teeth marks.

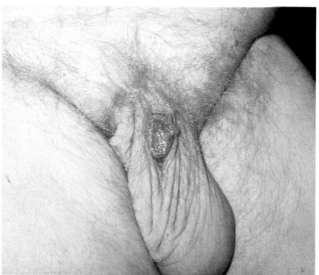

Fig. 25 Animal predator injury, in this case by a domestic dog, which was shut up for several days in a house with its owner who had died of coronary artery disease. The post-mortem depradations of animals, from ants to large mammals and reptiles in the tropics, can cause false alarms of criminal injury unless the doctor is aware of the possibility.

15

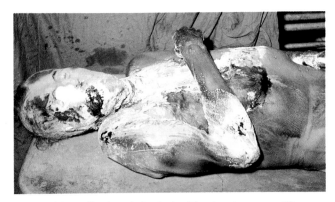

Fig. 26 Mummification of a body dead for almost one year. After absconding from a mental hospital, the victim hid in a hay-loft, which was warm and dry. When death took place from natural causes, this environment prevented the usual wet putrefaction. The skin became brown and leathery and the exposed surfaces were covered in mould. Though more common in hot, dry climates, it can occur in temperate zones, given unusual environmental conditions.

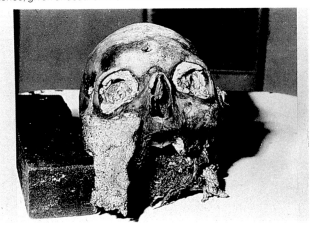

Fig. 27 Where death takes place in water or in very damp conditions, the usual putrefaction may be partly replaced by 'adipocere', where the subcutaneous fat is hydrolysed to waxy material which may retain the shape of the tissues for many years. This skull, recovered from the sea three months after death, shows adipocere of the orbital and buccal fat. Incidentally, identification was made by the presence of acromegaly, an old penetrating wound of the forehead and radiographic comparison of the frontal sinuses with previous hospital X-rays.

The pattern of injuries and death from road traffic accidents varies from country to country, with vehicle occupants being more frequent victims in advanced countries with a higher traffic density. However, world-wide the pedestrian is statistically the most vulnerable.

In pedestrians, the injuries can be conveniently classified into 'primary' and 'secondary' depending on whether they were caused by the direct impact of the vehicle or from being thrown to the ground. The mechanics of a pedestrian being lifted up on to a motor car are complex and do not always follow the theoretical pattern. However, it is useful in the reconstruction of an unwitnessed accident, if the medical examiner can attempt to interpret the various injuries.

This also applies to cyclists, motor-cyclists and the occupants of motor vehicles. The medico-legal consequences of a motor accident may be profound, both in relation to possible criminal charges against a reckless driver or to civil compensation and insurance matters, which may involve very large amounts of money. The pathologist or other doctor examining the injured or dead victims, should be careful to retain any physical evidence, especially where the accident was a 'hit-and-run' type where the vehicle may need to be traced by the police. Paint flakes and glass fragments in wounds, oil smears, tyre marks and soiled and damaged clothing should all be retained for forensic laboratory examination. Blood or breath alcohol estimations should be obtained where possible and in the dead victim, blood or urine samples should be analysed if death occurred within 12-24 hours of the accident.

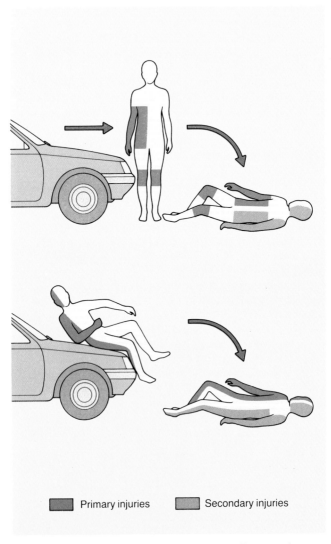

Primary injuries   Secondary injuries

Fig. 28 Types of injury sustained by pedestrians. These can be classified into primary (caused by direct impact of the vehicle) and secondary (due to subsequent falling or being thrown against the ground or other obstructions). In addition, the victim may be run over after falling, by either the same vehicle or another.

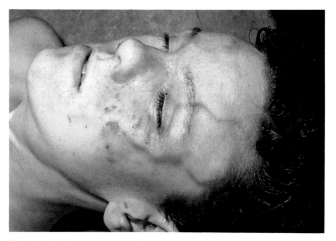

Fig. 29 Marks on the face of a pedestrian victim from the tread of a motor tyre. Whether in the unconscious live patient or the dead victim, it is essential that the doctor should record, measure and if possible, photograph such injuries. In a 'hit-and-run' accident, the police may be able to confirm the identity of the suspect vehicle by comparison with the tyre tread, as in this case where a truck was involved.

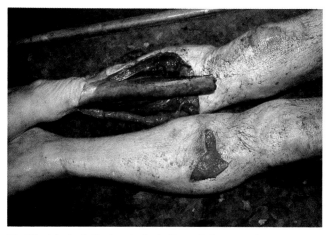

Fig. 30 Injuries to the legs typical of impact of a car against a pedestrian. Sometimes called a 'bumper fracture', the compound break of the tibia on one side and the laceration on the other, are due to primary impact of the fender of the vehicle. The doctor should always measure the height of the lesions above heel level, as this may help to confirm the identity of the vehicle in a 'hit-and-run' accident.

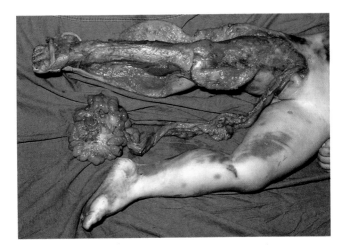

Fig. 31 A 'flaying injury' in a child run over by a bus. The stripping of the skin and underlying tissues from the limb is typical of a rotatory action of a large wheel which has also caused the friction abrasion on the opposite leg. The abdomen has also been run over, causing extrusion of the intestines through the torn perineum.

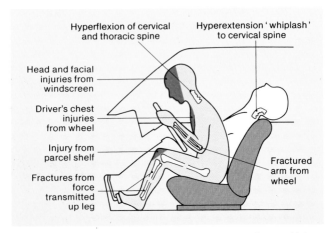

Fig. 32 Mechanism of injury in front-seat occupants of a car which suffers a frontal impact (80% of vehicle crashes). If not wearing a seat-belt, the body moves forwards, the legs strike the lower facia, the head strikes or penetrates the wind-screen and in the case of the driver, the chest may impact upon the wheel. Fractures of the arms and legs may occur from transmitted force up the tensed limbs.

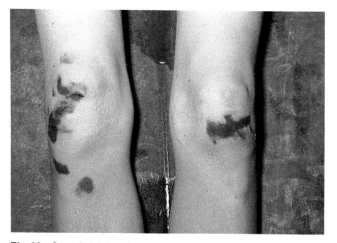

Fig. 33 Superficial abrasions on the knees of a front-seat passenger in a car which has been involved in a deceleration impact. The body, if unrestrained by a seat belt, slides forwards and the knees strike the parcel shelf. In former times, when cars had solid wooden instrument panels, similar but more severe injuries were called 'dash-board fractures'.

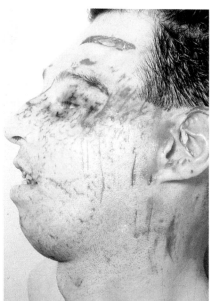

Fig. 34 Another typical deceleration injury, this time in an unrestrained driver. The numerous lacerations on the face, often triangular or stellate, are due to fragments of shattered toughened glass from the wind-screen. The horizontal laceration on the forehead, which overlies a fractured skull and brain damage, was caused by the upper metal rim of the wind-screen.

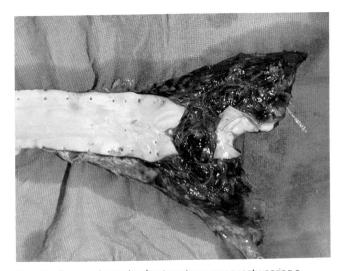

Fig. 35 Ruptured aorta in a front-seat passenger not wearing a seat-belt. The usual point of tearing is where the descending arch is attached to the front of the dorsal spine. The mechanism is usually a severe hyperextension-flexion movement ('whip-lash') caused by the head and shoulders swinging forwards on impact. Sometimes, this injury can occur as a result of the heart swinging violently within the thorax on impact, though then the point of tearing is often nearer the aortic valve.

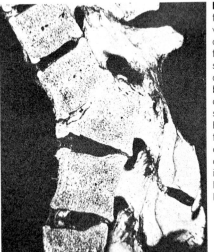

Fig. 36 Crush fracture of a thoracic vertebra of a car driver following a frontal impact. He survived for a considerable time, but there was complete loss of spinal cord function below the site of fracture, due to distortion of the spinal canal. This type of injury is preventable by a diagonal seat-belt.

Wounds

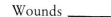

Wounds are usually classified according to whether or not they penetrate the skin, cause bleeding under the skin, or are caused by an incising object. These are called respectively 'abrasions', 'lacerations', 'contusions' or 'incised wounds'. Abrasions tend to display the pattern of the causative object most clearly, although often superficial bruising may also leave a clear imprint in the dermis. It is essential that the medical examiner should record any obvious pattern in a wound, as it may assist in identifying the weapon or other agent. A colour photograph is ideal, but monochrome photography or an accurate sketch may be very useful, in addition to a written description with exact measurements recorded.

As with all medical reports meant for use by lay persons such as police, lawyers or courts, non-technical language should be used in the description of wounds. 'Contusions' are 'bruises', 'abrasions' may be 'scratches' and 'lacerations' are 'cuts'. Medical jargon should be avoided wherever possible, unless there is no equivalent common word for a medical expression. Where medical terms are used, a brief explanation should be added.

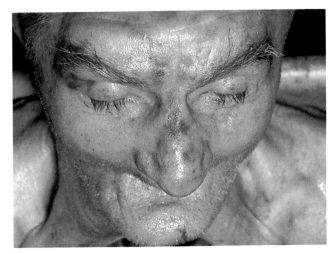

Fig. 37 Multiple superficial abrasions of the face, due to falling repeatedly on rough ground. Abrasions, also called 'grazes', are the most superficial of wounds, where the full thickness of the skin is not broken. However, pure abrasions are commonly mixed with deeper injury in which the dermal papillae are damaged, so that some bleeding occurs.

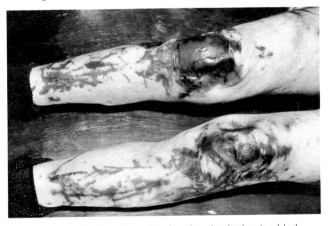

Fig. 38 Extensive abrasions of the legs in a drunk who stumbled unclothed amongst furniture before suffering a fractured skull. After death, abrasions may become dark and leathery due to drying of the damaged epidermis.

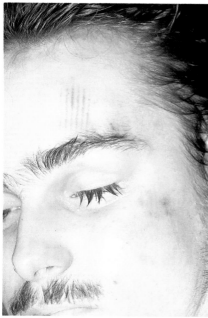

Fig. 39 Abrasions exhibit the pattern of the injuring object better than bruises or lacerations. This swimming-bath attendant found drowned, had facial abrasions which exactly matched the pattern of ridged tiles at the edge of the bath. It is essential to record, draw or photograph any patterned injuries on a victim.

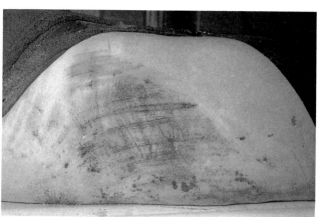

Fig. 40 Parallel lines of grazes or 'brush abrasions' typical of contact with a rough surface. These may be caused by friction of the body against the ground, as in the common 'gravel rash' of road accidents - or by a tangential impact by a weapon or vehicle. In this case, the abrasions were post-mortem, sustained when a murdered woman was dropped down a mine shaft.

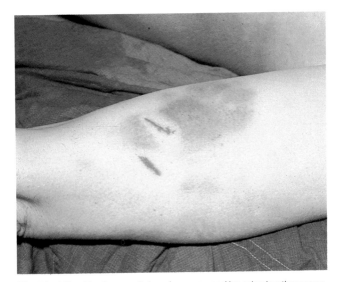

Fig. 41 Mixed bruises and abrasions, caused by gripping the upper arm during an assault. The small scratches are probably due to finger-nails. There was no bleeding, as bruises or 'contusions' are sub-cutaneous and these pure abrasions did not penetrate the epidermis.

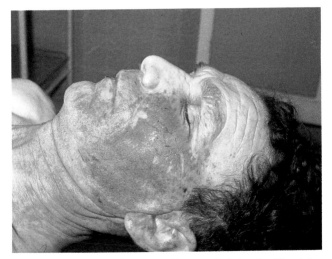

Fig. 42 Bruising of the face caused by repeated slapping. The victim was a night-watchman, tied up and assaulted by intruders.

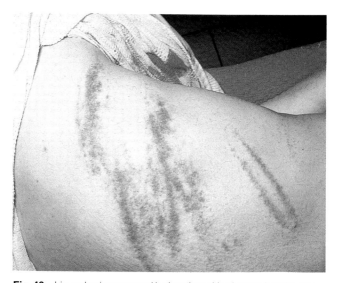

Fig. 43   Linear bruises caused by beating with a broom-handle. The injuries show a typical 'tram-line' pattern of two parallel lines. This is due to the impact of a circular or square rod, which compresses the central zone, so preventing capillary rupture, but stretches the tissues at each side causing sub-cutaneous haemorrhage.

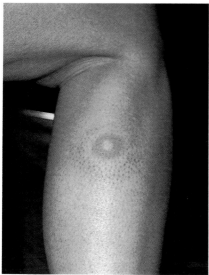

Fig. 44   Circular bruise with several zones of pallor, hyperaemia and contusion. This can only be due to the forcible impact of a spherical object, in this case a squash-ball.

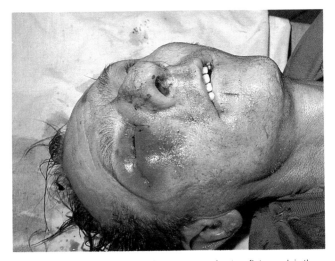

Fig. 45 A 'black eye' or orbital haematoma, due to a fist punch in the eye. There is associated abrasion of the upper cheek and nose. The following two illustrations indicate alternative mechanisms for a black eye, which must be borne in mind by the medical examiner.

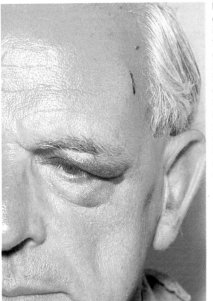

Fig. 46 A black eye caused by a trivial injury, seen on the temple. Due to gravity, blood beneath this injury flowed downwards over the course of a few hours and passed over the supra-orbital ridge into the orbit, causing haemorrhagic swelling of the eyelids.

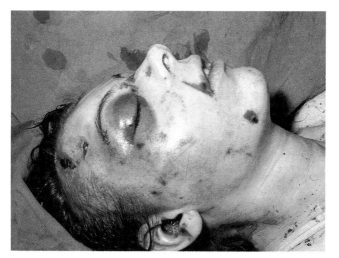

Fig. 47 The third mechanism of a black eye is a fractured base of skull. Following a severe head injury, blood from the subdural space entered the orbit through cracks in the floor of the anterior fossa and appeared in the eyelids.

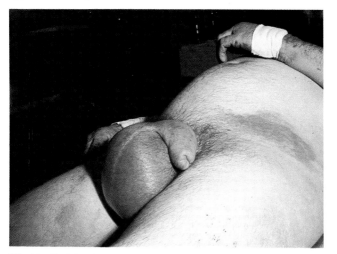

Fig. 48 Bruising. Haematoma of the scrotum (haematocele) associated with bruising in the right iliac fossa. These were caused by violent kicking during a gang fight, when the victim was lying on the ground. Death was due to intra-peritoneal bleeding from laceration of the mesentery.

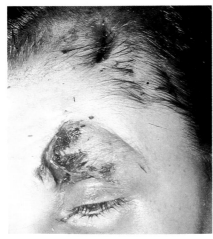

Fig. 49 Lacerations. Injury to the eyebrow and scalp caused by assault with a brick. The full thickness of the skin is penetrated – an essential part of a laceration, which therefore bleeds copiously. Over the scalp and eyebrow ridge, the skin splits on impact, being supported beneath by bone. Gravitational bleeding into the orbit has already begun.

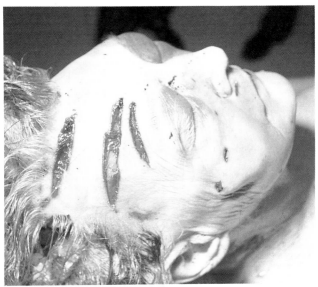

Fig. 50 Lacerations. Multiple lacerations of the scalp inflicted with a metal bar during robbery (see Fig. 2). Thought at first by the police to be knife or axe wounds, the clean-cut appearance is again typical of splitting of the scalp by a blunt instrument due to the underlying support by bone. However, close examination reveals that the edges of the wounds are crushed and that tissue bridges survive within the wounds.

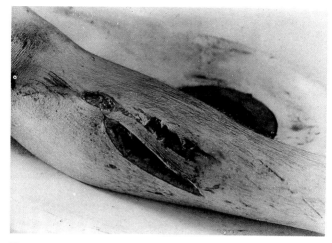

Fig. 51 Incised wounds. Slashes from a knife sustained by a victim of a hooligan attack. Unlike stabs, slashed wounds are longer than they are deep. External bleeding is the main danger to life, rather than deep visceral damage.

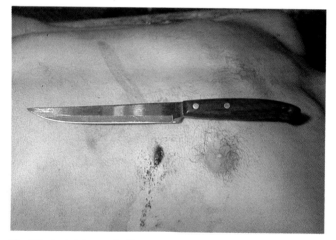

Fig. 52 Incised wounds. The stab wound is deeper than it is wide and an externally trivial injury is often fatal. The wound may be slightly smaller than the width of the knife, as shown here. This is due to gaping of the wound and the elasticity of the tissues drawing the ends of wound together.

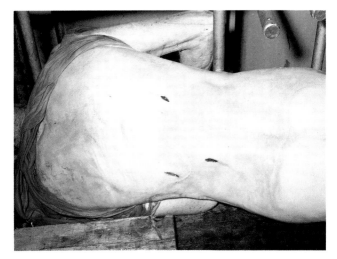

Fig. 53 Incised wounds. Multiple stab wounds with the same knife as in fig. 52, showing variation in size. 'Rocking' of the knife enlarges the wounds, as seen on the left side of the body. With a tapering blade, the depth of penetration also determines the size of the wound. In Fig. 3 the effect of twisting the knife is seen.

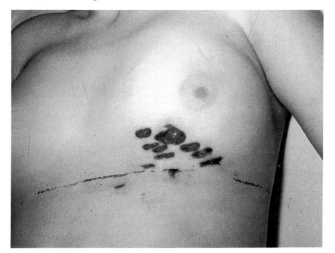

Fig. 54 Incised wounds. Multiple stabs below the breast of a woman. Some overlie each other, making it difficult to determine the exact number of injuries. Such wounds have a sadistic sexual content, as do those on the lower abdomen, buttocks and perineum.

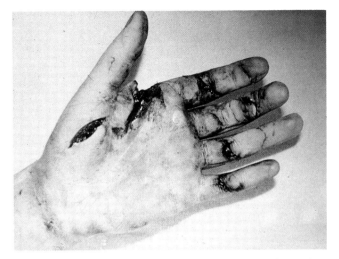

Fig. 55 Incised wounds. Typical 'defence wounds' in a knife attack. In an attempt to ward off the weapon, wounds have been sustained in the angle between thumb and first finger and on the hypothenar eminence. Grasping of the blade has caused cuts across the flexor surface of the inter-phalangeal joints.

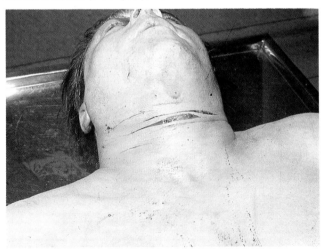

Fig. 56 Incised wounds. Suicidal cut-throat attempt. There are several classical 'tentative incisions', which are the hallmark of self-infliction. The deceased abandoned the attempt and killed himself by jumping from a height.

33

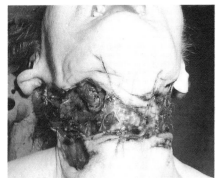

Fig. 57 Suicidal throat wound. In spite of the extensive damage, the self-inflicted nature of this wound is shown by tentative cuts, even though some are at right angles.

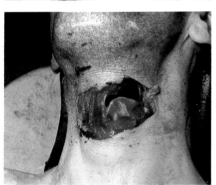

Fig. 58 Homicidal throat wound. There are no tentative incisions and the jagged wound is deep. It is not possible, however, to be sure of murder merely because of the absence of trial cuts.

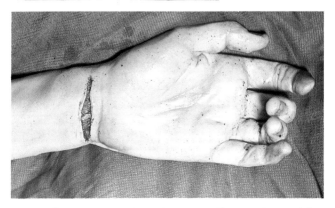

Fig. 59 Classical cut wrist in suicide gesture. The injury is on the left side, usual with most right-handed people. Such a wound is rarely fatal, as the tendency to hyper-extend the wrist causes the radial artery to shelter against the head of the radius.

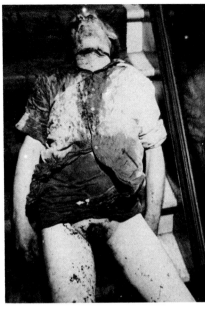

Fig. 60 Self-inflicted injuries. The deceased has removed his genitals, cut his throat through a full circle and punctured both eyeballs, all with blunt scissors. Though the police suspected murder, the picture is typical of self-mutilation associated with mental disorder, in this case paranoid and religious delusions.

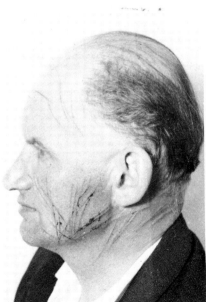

Fig. 61 Self-inflicted injuries. Here the motive was gain, in that the victim attempted to simulate robbery with violence, to cover his theft of his employer's money. The superficial, regular, parallel scratches, which avoid the sensitive regions of eyes, nose, lips and ears, are obviously self-inflicted.

Firearm wounds

The medical aspects of gun-shot wounds depend largely upon the type of weapon used, especially whether a smooth-bore shot-gun or a rifled weapon such as a revolver, semi-automatic pistol or an automatic weapon, (usually military) has been used.

A shot-gun discharges a large number of small shot in a shallow divergent cone, so that the wound pattern varies according to the range. The single projectile from a rifled weapon offers much less evidence of range, except at contact or very close distances.

All guns produce characteristic effects at point-blank range, due to the flame and gas from the muzzle. In older weapons and ammunition, especially shot-guns, smoke and unburnt powder add to the soiling of skin or clothing.

Some modern shot-gun cartridges contain plastic cups which open out during flight and produce recognisable marks on the skin at close range, sometimes in the form of a cross.

In all gun-shot wounds, radiology should be performed to detect metallic foreign bodies in the tissues. Any bullets, shot, wads or metallic fragments found at operation of autopsy, should be carefully preserved and handed to the police for specialist examination. After death, soiled clothing or skin should also be retained, for laboratory chemical examination for the identification of propellant and primer residues.

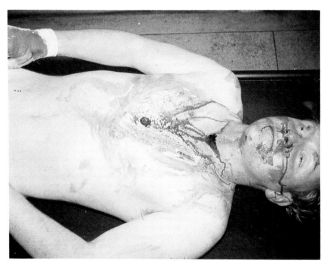

Fig. 62 A very close-range discharge of a .410 shot-gun into the chest. Clothing has prevented the skin from being burnt or soiled by powder. The wound is round and small, with no satellite pellet marks. The wads were in the wound. The direction of the blood flow indicates that the victim lay on his back with his head low, after being injured.

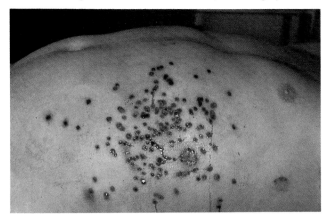

Fig. 63 A gun-shot wound from a 12-bore shotgun at about eight metres range. The spread of pellets is about 20-24 cm but in addition, there is a circular bruise at the lower left centre due to the impact of the cartridge wad. The roughly circular pattern indicates that the weapon was fired at right angles to the body surface. By courtesy of Dr. O. G. Williams.

37

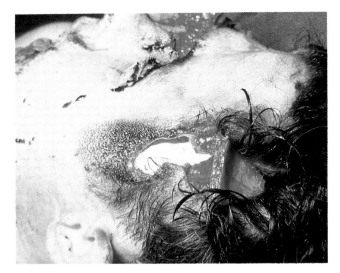

Fig. 64 A contact 12-bore shot-gun wound in the temple. The skin shows black powder residue, indicating both a close discharge and also an oblique angle, as the powder mark is elliptical.

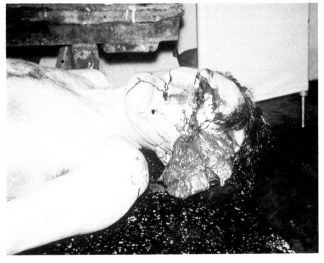

Fig. 65 A suicidal discharge of a shot-gun into the mouth. This is one of the three main sites of election for self-destruction, the others being the temple (Fig. 64) and the chest. Shot-guns produce an exit wound in the head or limb, but rarely penetrate the thorax or abdomen.

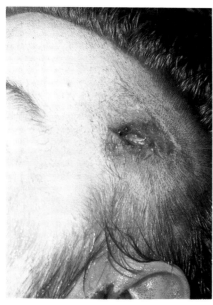

Fig. 66 Near-contact discharge of an automatic pistol, showing reddening and burning around the wound. There are no smoke or powder marks, due to the clean propellant used. This entrance wound shows everted edges and is split due to the rebound of gases from the underlying skull.

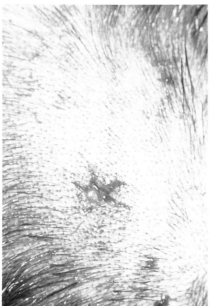

Fig. 67 Exit wound of a revolver bullet on the scalp. The wound is stellate and everted and the lack of any burning or soiling eliminates the possibility of it being an entrance wound.

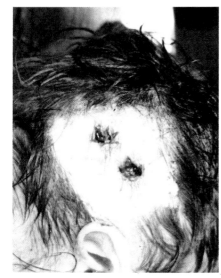

Fig. 68 Two .22 rifle bullet exit wounds on the head of a child. Again the typical stellate, everted appearance is seen, with no soiling or burning. Over bone, such as on the scalp, a contact entrance wound can be stellate and everted due to rupture of a gas blister from the muzzle.

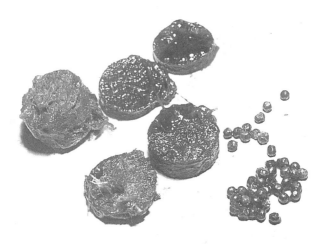

Fig. 69 Wads and shot from a 12-bore shot-gun wound. The wads may travel 2-6 metres to lodge in the wound, assisting in the estimation of range. Pellets should be retained for forensic examination to identify the cartridge type. Modern ammunition may contain plastic cups etc., which can cause additional surface injuries.

Burns

The most common types of fatal burns are those sustained in fires in buildings, where considerable destruction of the tissues may occur. In these circumstances, a major medico-legal necessity is to determine whether the victim was dead or alive during the fire, as many attempts to conceal a homicide have been made in this way. The two main criteria are the presence of soot in the deep airways and the presence of carbon monoxide in the blood. It must be noted that although carboxy-haemoglobin is a reliable marker of respiration after the onset of the fire, the converse is not true and many authenticated instances are on record of undoubted life during a fire, with no absorbtion of monoxide. This may be especially so where there is rapid flash fire, as sometimes in vehicles where gasoline is involved.

The differentiation of ante-mortem from post-mortem burns is also important, but extremely difficult where the burns have been sustained very near the moment of death. Hyperaemia of the margin of the burn is not a reliable indicator, as it can occur from heat applied many minutes after death has taken place. Histological evidence of a cellular vital reaction is the only safe indication of ante-mortem burning.

In electrocution, an appreciation of basic physics is necessary to understand the effects upon the body. There must be a pathway for a current and to produce fatal ventricular fibrillation, this current must attain at least 50 milliamperes across the chest for several seconds. The current depends upon both the applied voltage and the skin resistance, which explains the greater danger in wet conditions when skin resistance is greatly reduced.

The pathway is usually from a hand touching a live conductor to earth, either through the feet to ground or via the other hand to an earthed contact or to a conductor at a lower potential. Most deaths are due to cardiac arrest from the direct effects of the current, but a few are caused by paralysis or spasm of the thoracic and diaphragmatic respiratory muscles, in which case the victim will be cyanosed, as opposed to pallid from cardiac arrest.

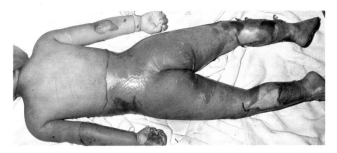

Fig. 70 Wet burns or 'scalds' on an infant who was accidentally left for a few minutes in a hot bath. Death occurred a few days later from bronchopneumonia. The surface area involved is critical, survival being unlikely if a third to a half is involved in a child - and much less with advancing age.

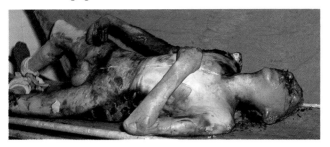

Fig. 71 Extensive burning in a house fire, showing the 'pugilistic attitude' of limb flexion and spinal opisthotonus due to heat contracture of the muscles. The burns were post-mortem, death being due to prior carbon monoxide poisoning from fumes.

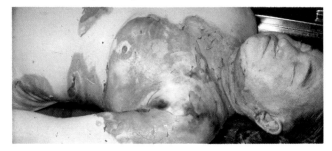

Fig. 72 If sustained at, or around the moment of death, it can be difficult or impossible to differentiate ante- from post-mortem burns. Most of these, caused by burning clothing, were probably ante-mortem as shown by the bright red margin, but this is not a reliable sign, as a heat blister is seen on undamaged skin.

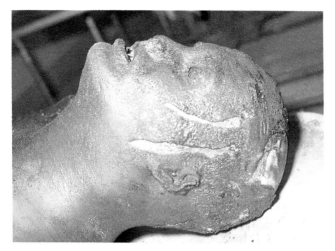

Fig. 73 Splitting of the scalp due to heat contraction of the skin. These were at first mistaken for knife wounds by police. On the top of the head, deep burning had caused a spurious 'extra-dural haematoma' inside the skull, again sometimes confused with ante-mortem violence.

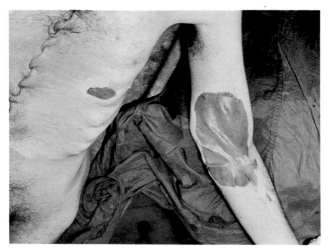

Fig. 74 Unmistakable post-mortem burn, due to a hot water bottle being applied to the chest with the arm folded across it, in an attempt to revive a dead person. The sharp margin between leathery epidermis and the intact skin is characteristic.

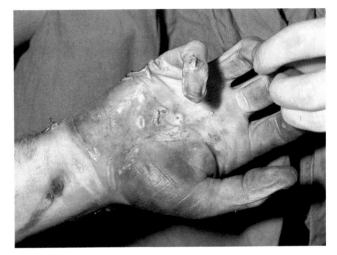

Fig. 75 Hand of an electrician, showing multiple spark burns and collapsed blisters from prolonged contact with mains voltage. The linear lesion in the wrist is more thermal in nature.

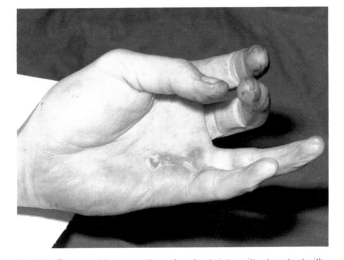

Fig. 76 Two spark burns on the palm, due to intermittent contact with a faulty electric drill. The lesions show a pale areola around a brown nodule of fused keratin. In fatalities, there must be both an entrance point and an exit to earth for sufficient current (at least 50 milliamps) to flow across the chest and cause cardiac arrest or respiratory paralysis.

44

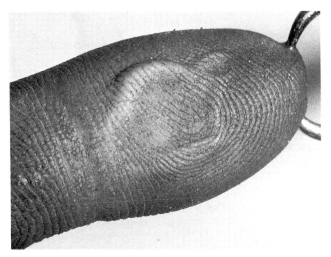

Fig. 77 A firm contact with a conductor carrying 240 volts AC. The finger tip shows two collapsed blisters caused by the heating effect of the current. This lesion or a single small spark burn may be the only signs of electrocution and must be searched for diligently where the possibility exists.

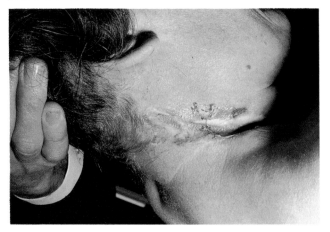

Fig. 78 A presumed suicide, but possibly a homicide, by electricity. The wire wrapped around the neck has left a typical electrical mark with a pale zone and peeling of the epidermis.

Cold and neglect

Hypothermia can occur in temperate climates and is relatively common in European winters. It mostly affects the old and young and is sometimes related to neglect in other aspects. Where the body temperature drops to 28° Centrigrade or less, recovery is unlikely. There may be no external or internal signs, but where these are present, the most common include a dusky-pink discoloration of the skin, mainly over joints and extensor surfaces, rarely with blistering. Internally, acute gastric erosions are the most common indicators, as well as fat necrosis of the pancreas. Frank frostbite of the extremities is rare except in extreme conditions.

Neglect also occurs most often in the very old and young, the former usually being self-inflicted. Poor hygiene, dirty clothing, verminous hair and skin and nutritional deficiencies are common. In starved infants, a wizened, aged facial appearance may be seen, together with dehydration and a concave abdomen. Internally, apart from general wasting, there may be empty intestines filled with gas and a dilated gall-bladder due to lack of food stimulus to emptying.

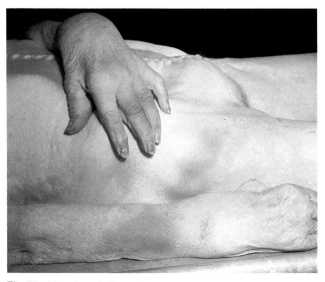

Fig. 79 Hypothermia. Brownish-pink discoloration of the skin over joints and extensor surfaces, in this case the hip and forearm. Knees and shins are also often involved. The cause for the colour change is not clear, but is partly due to failure of the cooled tissues to dissociate oxy-haemoglobin. Sometimes actual skin blistering may occur.

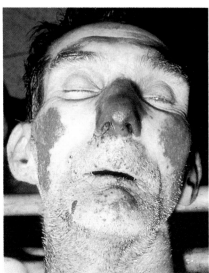

Fig. 80 Hypothermia. Lesions due to cold may affect more protruberant areas of the body, such as the nose, cheeks or digits. Here the effect upon the face has been accentuated, as the victim had a pre-existing malar flush due to mitral stenosis. The hypothermia developed in bed, but in an unheated bedroom.

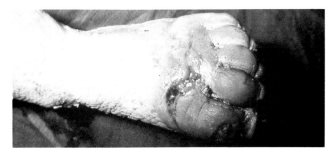

Fig. 81 Neglect. Hypothermia in an infant which has progressed to actual frost-bite, with necrosis and sloughing of the distal part of the foot. The child was left in a urine-soaked cot in an unheated farmhouse. When death occurred, it was placed in a sack with a brick and dropped down a well.

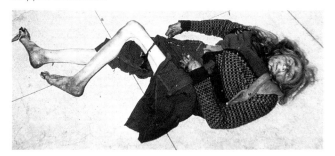

Fig. 82 An old woman who died of hypothermia and malnutrition, though poverty was not a factor. The external signs of hypothermia were confined to the feet, but internal evidence comprised fat necrosis in the pancreas and acute gastric erosions.

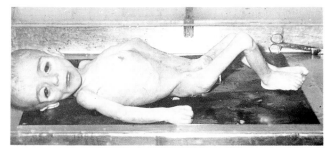

Fig. 83 This infant was grossly emaciated, with a scaphoid abdomen, Hippocratic facies and sunken eyes. Internally, the intestines were devoid of food and contained only gas. The child had been deliberately starved by the parents.

Asphyxia

Modern concepts of 'asphyxia' have reduced the reliance upon the old classical signs of congestion and petechial haemorrhages. It is recognised that especially in cases of pressure around the neck, such congestive appearances are due to obstructed venous return, rather than to hypoxia. Sub-pleural petechiae, the so-called 'Tardieu spots', are also far less specific that was once thought and can be found to some degree in almost all autopsies, especially near the hilum and in the fissures of the lungs. Pressure on the neck rarely causes effective constriction of the trachea or larynx and airway obstruction is usually due to raising of the tongue against the palate. The petechiae in the eyelids, conjunctivae, facial skin and the bleeding from ears and nose in strangulation is mainly due to jugular compression. Many deaths from pressure on the neck are rapid and not accompanied by congestive-haemorrhagic signs but are due to cardiac arrest from pressure upon the carotid body or sheath, leading to a vagal reflex which causes bradycardia or even immediate cardiac arrest.

In suffocation, such as the envelopment of the head in a plastic bag, death may also be very rapid and often unaccompanied by congestive signs, the mechanism being obscure - a similar situation to the sudden deaths which can occur when a person enters an irrespirable atmosphere such as carbon dioxide or nitrogen.

Strangulation, either manually or by ligature and hanging, may present either as 'classical' congestive asphyxia, where death must have taken at least half a minute or usually longer to occur - or to 'vagal inhibition', which may be instantaneous or supervene at any time, whether or not congestive changes have had time to become apparent.

The so-called 'traumatic asphyxia' presents the most gross congestive-haemorrhagic appearances, due to fixation of the chest and strenuous efforts to inspire.

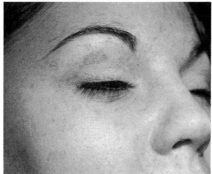

Fig. 84 Manual pressure around the neck has produced a shower of fine petechial haemorrhages in the upper eyelids. There were more sparse petechiae around the lips and the rest of the face above the neck. These haemorrhages are caused more by obstruction of venous return than by anoxia.

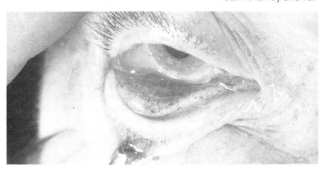

Fig. 85 Haemorrhages inside the lower lid in manual strangulation. They may also occur on the sclera of the eyeball itself, and may be present when no petechiae are visible on the facial skin.

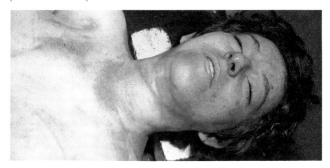

Fig. 86 Traumatic asphyxia. In this poorly-named syndrome, death is due to fixation of the chest by external pressure. In this case, the victim was crushed in a crowd, causing congestion and confluent petechial haemorrhages in the neck and face, especially the eyelids and conjunctivae. Areas of bruising are present on the upper chest.

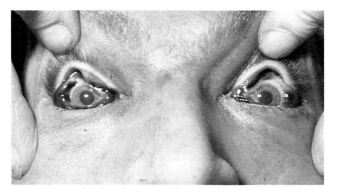

Fig. 87 Traumatic asphyxia. Gross conjunctival haemorrhages bulging through the lids, due to fixation of the chest by an overturned tractor. The face is congested and covered in tiny petechial haemorrhages, which extend down to the thoracic inlet, a typical level of demarcation in traumatic asphyxia. The congestion and bleeding are largely due to futile attempts to inspire against a fixed thoracic cage, rather than to pure anoxia.

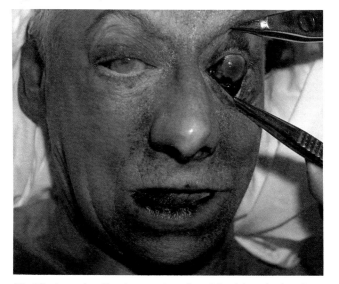

Fig. 88 Inversion. The deceased was found dead, hanging head downwards out of bed, after a heavy drinking bout. His posture together with his acute alcoholic poisoning, at least partially prevented respiratory movements of the chest, though it is impossible to say how much of the gross congestion and haemorrhage is post-mortem.

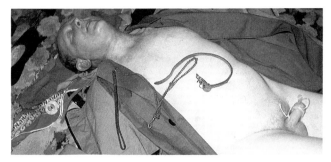

Fig. 89 Masochistic 'asphyxia'. Self-strangulation with a dog collar and lead (removed) during a sexual exercise. There was rubber fetishism, including masks and partial transvestism. The death was variously ascribed to suicide and even homicide, but the sexual features indicate that it was accidental.

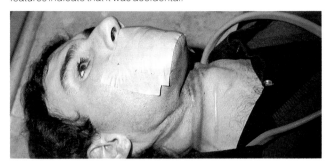

Fig. 90 Masochistic 'asphyxia'. Self-hanging with an electric cable, with features that indicate a masochistic motive, rather than suicidal. The face is gagged and the wrists and ankles were chained, indicating a perverse desire for restraint. Death was not asphyxial, but due to cardiac arrest from sudden pressure on the neck, as demonstrated by the pallor of the face and lack of petechiae.

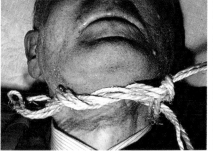

Fig. 91 Suicidal hanging with thick cord suspended from a staircase. There is gross congestion and cyanosis above the cord, contrasting with the pale skin below, indicating that death was not sudden, there being sufficient time for venous occlusion to become apparent.

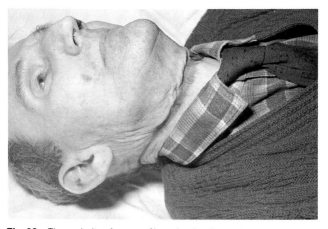

Fig. 92 The majority of cases of hanging lead to rapid, virtually instantaneous death from cardiac arrest due to sudden impact upon the carotid vessels. Here the face is pale, with no congestion nor 'asphyxial' signs. The rising ligature mark is obvious: after a short post-mortem interval, the mark appears to be brown and leathery, due to drying of the damaged epidermis.

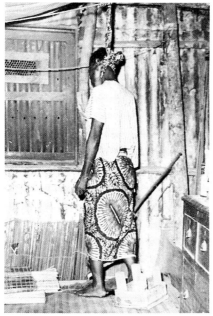

Fig. 93 There need be no free suspension of the body to achieve hanging. Here the feet are flat on the floor and many hangings have taken place from door knobs or chairs, the partial weight of the body being sufficient to cause pressure on the neck.

53

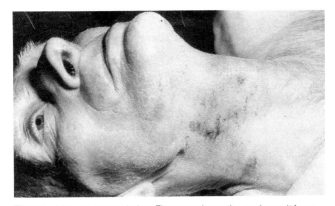

Fig. 94 Manual strangulation. Fingermarks on the neck result from pressure and abrasion of the assailant's fingers. Although over-interpretation should be avoided, the more prominent marks over the right angle of the jaw can be accepted as thumb impressions from a right-handed assailant. Many of the marks are small abrasions, rather than bruises and are likely to have been caused by fingernails. Note that the face is pale and that there are no petechial haemorrhages in the eyes, lips or facial skin, indicating that death was not 'congestive' or 'asphyxial', but due to rapid cardiac arrest from pressure on the carotid structures.

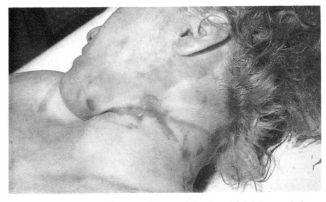

Fig. 95 A ligature mark around the neck in a homicidal strangulation. The ligature was a wide folded scarf, but when pulled tight, the bands of tension leave narrow marks on the skin. The cross-over point can be seen. The face and neck above the mark are congested and there were petechiae in the eyes, indicating that death was not the sudden 'cardiac arrest' type.

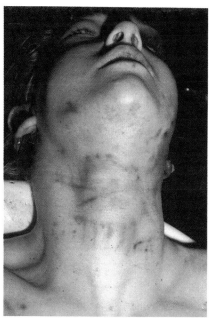

Fig. 96 Manual strangulation. The row of vertical scratches on the lower part of the front of the neck and the corresponding abrasions over the larynx are due to the victim struggling to tear away the constricting hand, whilst the marks around the jaw are from the killer. In contrast to Fig. 94 there are signs of a congestive death, such as bleeding from the ear and nose and punctate haemorrhages in the face and eyelids.

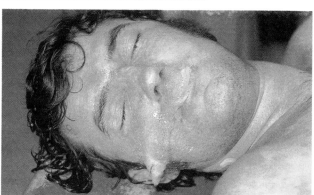

Fig. 97 Drowning. The copious froth, often slightly tinged with blood, is indicative of drowning. Although pulmonary oedema from natural causes, such as the left ventricular failure of hypertensive heart disease may produce froth, it is seldom blood-stained and, of course, the surrounding circumstances are most relevant. In drowning the froth rapidly disperses and the medical examiner may not find it either externally or even internally if there is any appreciable post-mortem interval.

Head injury

This is a most important topic in forensic medicine, both in accidental deaths and in assault and homicide. The various types of meningeal haemorrhage and their relationship to skull fracture and blunt trauma should be clearly understood. The recognition of **contre coup** lesions in differentiating a blow upon a fixed head from a passive fall is of considerable use in interpreting unwitnessed injuries. The various types of black eye are important, as misinterpretation of a scalp wound or fractured base of skull as a direct blow to the face can have unfortunate legal consequences.

Injuries to the scalp are also confused by some medical examiners as well as police officers: an apparently sharply-cut wound may be due to blunt trauma, as an injury over the underlying support of the skull may split cleanly and appear to be an incised wound from a sharp weapon. The differentiation depends upon experience, aided by a close inspection of the wound. A blunt split will show marginal bruising, tissue bridges in the depths of the wound and sometimes intact hairs crossing the wound.

The types of skull fracture require classification and where depressed or pond fractures occur, the focal nature of the impact should be recognised. A linear or comminuted fracture may occur at a point distant from the impact, where the distortion of the skull exceeds the elastic threshold of the bone.

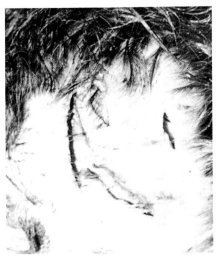

Fig. 98 Split wounds of the scalp inflicted with a blunt instrument (poker). They are sharply-cut, at first suggesting incised wounds, but the edges are slightly bruised (see also Fig. 50).

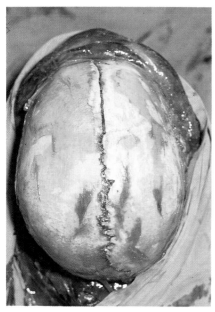

Fig. 99 Fracture of the skull in a young adult due to a fall from a height. Fractures occur when the deformation of a bone under stress exceeds its elastic threshold. In this case, the line of weakness is the relatively immature fusion of the interparietal suture line, which also extends into the position of the metopic suture between the frontal bones.

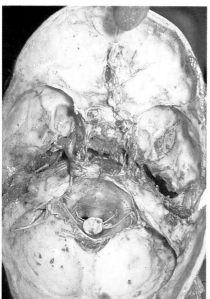

Fig. 100 Fractured base of skull in a 14-year-old pedestrian following a road accident. The impact due to a secondary injury caused by falling on to the temporal area, has caused a side-to-side fracture through the line of weakness in the skull base, passing anterior to the petrous temporal bones and through the pituitary fossa. X-ray of the head on admission to hospital revealed no fracture.

57

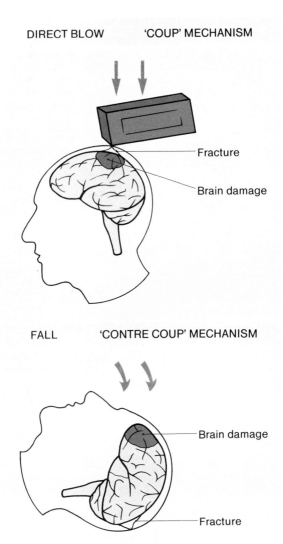

Fig. 101 The mechanism of 'coup' and 'contre coup' brain damage. When a fixed head is struck, the skull fracture (if present) and the cerebral bruising are on the same side, but where a falling head is abruptly decelerated by striking the ground, then brain damage is usually on the contra-lateral part of the brain. This may be of considerable use in differentiating a direct assault from a fall.

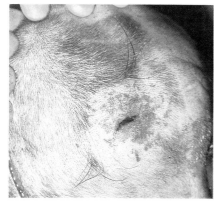

Fig. 102 A small occipito-parietal laceration in a victim of a drunken assault. The accused claimed that he had only pushed the deceased over, but the incident was unwitnessed. Autopsy (Fig. 103) helped to clarify the position.

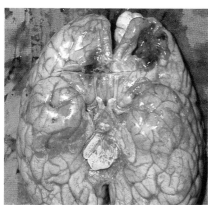

Fig. 103 The brain from the preceding case revealed cortical damage only in both frontal lobes, the classical contre coup injury from an occipital impact, This proved that the victim had not been struck on the head. In this case, there was a fracture of the left orbital plate, with bleeding into the eye socket on that side (see Fig. 47).

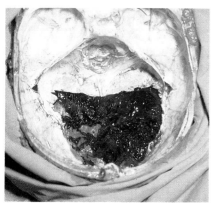

Fig. 104 An extra-dural haemorrhage following a blow to the head. About 85% of these lesions are associated with a skull fracture. This case is unusual in that the bleeding is in the posterior fossa, as the usual vessel to be damaged is the middle meningeal artery where it traverses the temporo-parietal area.

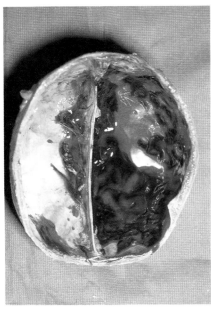

Fig. 105 An acute sub-dural haemorrhage following a head injury. There was no fracture of the skull. Sub-durals are most common in infancy and old age, but they can occur at all times of life. They are often unilateral but they are not reliable indicators of a contre coup mechanism.

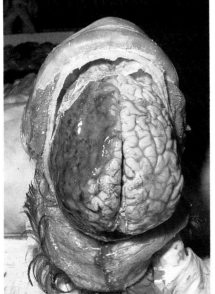

Fig. 106 A chronic sub-dural haematoma, regularly found in autopsies on old people. They may be symptomless or may have given rise to unilateral neurological signs or even mimicked senile dementia. They can be caused by trivial trauma to the head, which may not be recorded in the history of the case.

Infanticide and child abuse _____

The most important aspect of this topic is the total unreliability of most methods of attempting to determine live birth in a newly-born infant. The old 'old flotation tests' for autopsy samples of lungs are utterly unreliable and have been totally discredited by all modern authors. There is no valid way of differentiating lungs which have only taken a few breaths from the still-born lung, as even histology is unreliable, including the height of the bronchial epithelium. Where substantial respiration has occurred (in the absence of any putrefaction) gross inspection is probably as useful as any other method. Crepitation of pink aerated lung, especially at the lower margins, is the best criterion. The application of artificial respiration and active inflation of the lungs must also be considered. Where any doubt exists, the benefit of such doubt must be given in favour of a presumed stillbirth. Any significant degree of post-mortem change, with possible gas formation, always invalidates any opinion about live birth, unless there is food in the stomach or other accessory evidence of a separate existence. Even where live birth has been established, for a charge of infanticide to be brought, evidence must be found of an act of deliberate commission or omission which led to death. The latter is extremely difficult to prove. Caution must be used in commenting about the presence of the umbilical cord around the neck, as it may be there as an innocent obstetric complication or even become wrapped around the neck in post-mortem. Even ligatures around the neck are not always provable as the cause of death.

The child abuse syndrome, also known as the 'battered child' or 'non-accidental injury in childhood' syndrome is an important problem constituting a major aspect of paediatrics and pathology. The differentiation from simple accidents can be difficult, the hall-mark being repetition of bruises and fractures, characteristic radiological appearances, the occurrence of intracranial haemorrhages especially subdural haematomata, retinal and vitreous haemorrhages, intra-abdominal injury due to a ruptured viscus and more bizarre surface injuries such as bites, burns and patterned injuries.

The injuring parents or guardians usually offer a plausible explanation, which is, however, at variance with the nature and extent of the lesions, especially with the repetitive pattern. Bruises of varying ages and skeletal injuries in different stages of healing are particularly suspicious.

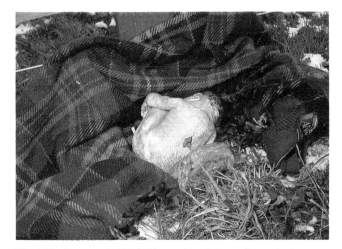

Fig. 107 A concealed birth. The newborn infant and attached placenta were dumped in a car rug on a lonely country road. The problem for the medical examiner is to differentiate between a still-birth and a live birth, as well as to investigate the possibility of infanticide.

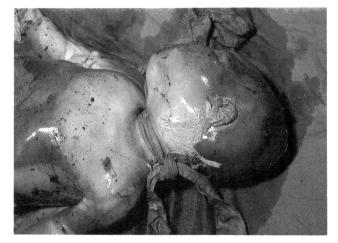

Fig. 108 A putrefied new-born with a tape tied around the neck. Although suspicious it could not be determined whether live birth had occurred, nor that the tape had caused death, as all autopsy findings were essentially negative.

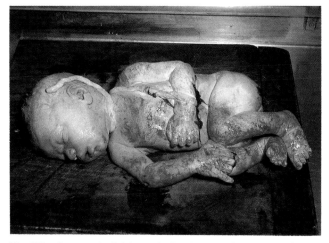

Fig. 109 A concealed birth, again showing no definite autopsy evidence of live birth or separate existence. The umbilical cord was wrapped around the neck, but this in itself is not necessarily suspicious, as it can occur spontaneously during parturition or during disposal of the body.

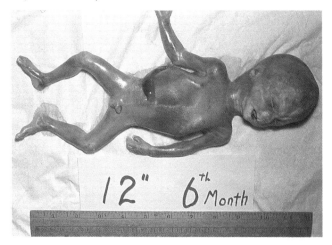

Fig. 110 Maturity of the fetus can be estimated with reasonable accuracy by measuring the crown-heel length. This aborted fetus of about six months gestation was 12 inches (30 cm) long. The general rule is that after the fourth month, the length of the fetus in centimetres is five times the gestation period in months, although there is considerable variation from case to case.

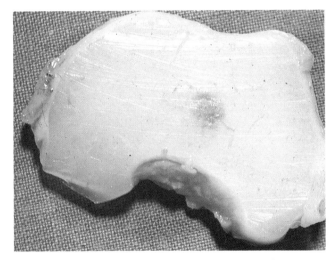

Fig. 111 Fetal maturity can be estimated by reference to the appearance of ossification centres in the skeleton. This centre in the lower end of the femur is a marker for full gestation, appearing around 40 weeks. Another of similar date is in the calcaneum. These can be detected either radiologically or by direct dissection.

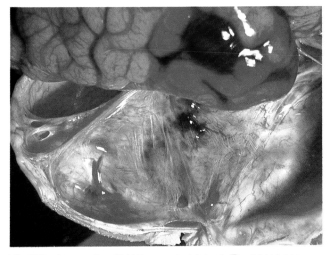

Fig. 112 A cause for still-birth or perinatal death. There has been tearing of the dural membranes (falx) with consequent meningeal haemorrhage, due to excessive moulding of the head during passage through the maternal canal.

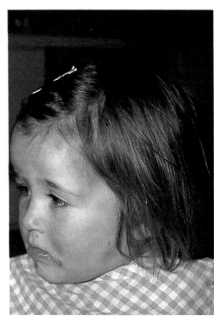

Fig. 113 Bruising of the forehead and lips in a live child. Any bruising, especially if multiple and of differing duration, is highly suspicious unless adequate explanation can be offered by the parents (see also Fig. 1). Where suspicion is strong, whole body radiography is advisable, as bruising and bone damage are the main diagnostic features of child abuse.

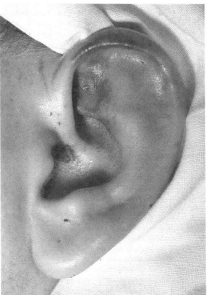

Fig. 114 A bruised ear in a small infant. Injuries of ears, eyes, lips and fingers are particularly suspicious. This child had a sub-dural haemorrhage and fractured skull from repeated head injuries.

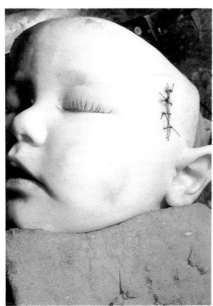

Fig. 115 A bite mark on the cheek of an infant. The two opposing semi-lunar bruises fitted the shape of the dental arches of an adult, although it was alleged by the parent that the family dog had bitten the child. It transpired that the mother was the culprit. The child died from a skull fracture and a burr-hole incision is seen, made to attempt drainage of a sub-dural haematoma, the most common cause of fatal child abuse.

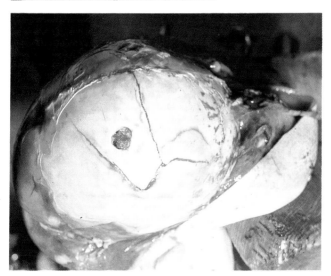

Fig. 116 A fissured fracture of the skull in an infant, who was thrown against the floor by a parent. A surgical burr-hole has been made to drain the frequent lesion, a subdural haemorrhage.

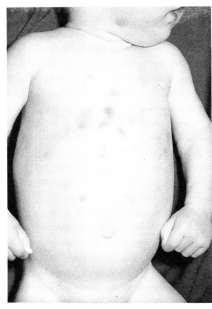

Fig. 117 Bruises on the chest and abdomen of an infant, typical of the discoid marks made by adult finger-tips. The child was prodded by a male guardian whilst the mother was absent, because he became irritated at the infant's crying. It rapidly became moribund and died on admission to hospital (see Fig 118).

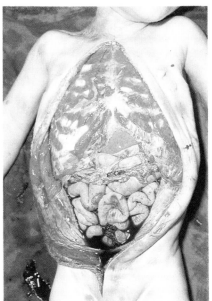

Fig. 118 At autopsy on the child shown in Fig. 117, extensive intra-abdominal bleeding was found, due to a rupture of the liver. Damage to an abdominal viscus (intestine or liver) is, after head injuries, the next most common cause of death in battered children.

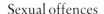

In both the living and dead, it is essential to make a full general examination, as well as concentrating upon the genital area. Especially where the woman has been previously accustomed to intercourse, or where intercourse has commenced with consent, there may be minimal or absent signs on the perineum: other marks such as bites, scratches and bruises on other parts of the body may have more evidential value of sexual activity.

The clothing should be seen, for evidence of tearing or foreign material, such as vegetation if the assault was said to have occurred outdoors. Pressure marks on the shoulders, buttocks, thighs and calves may also substantiate forcible holding against the ground, especially if there are focal injuries from stones, twigs etc.

The examination of the genitalia should be left until last, especially in the living. In a fatal case of rape and murder, it is unwise for the medical examiner to use the rectum or vagina for temperature estimations at the scene, because of the danger of contaminating a later examination for semen. If a temperature is needed, the mouth or axilla should be used with appropriate correction for a slightly lower temperature.

Swabs of the perieum, anus, vulva, mid-vagina and fornices should be taken before any further digital examination or dissection is undertaken.

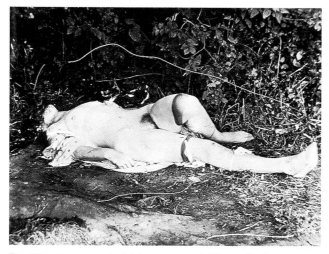

Fig. 119 The scene of a fatal sexual assault. The medical examiner must evaluate posture, disordered clothing, general injuries, genital damage and preserve trace evidence, which may include fibres, vegetation, hairs, seminal and blood stains etc. The same considerations apply as in the examination of live victims, with the added complications of the fatal injuries.

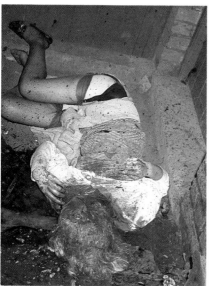

Fig. 120 Sexual assaults and attempted rape may be accompanied by gross violence, often precipitated by refused or withdrawn consent to intercourse or by taunting over lack of sexual prowess. The degree of violence accompanying sexual arousal may be extreme, as in this case of head injury.

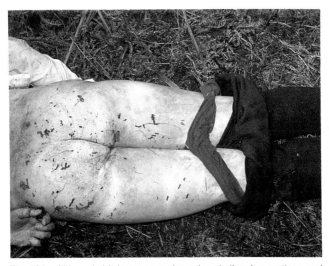

Fig. 121 Although this is a rape and murder, similar observations and investigations must be made in live victims where the circumstances dictate. Here the rolled-down knickers and trousers are obvious: the debris on the buttocks would have confirmed pressure against vegetation if a live victim had been examined elsewhere. The bleeding from the perineum comes from genital trauma.

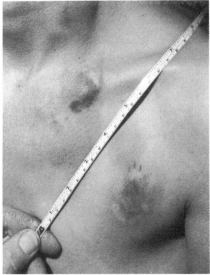

Fig. 122 Extra-genital injury must always be sought during examination, especially as it may be of considerable value on occasions where no damage has been caused to the vulval area. In this live victim of a multiple rape, obvious bite marks are seen on the breast and neck. Dental examination and swabs for saliva grouping should be considered in such cases.

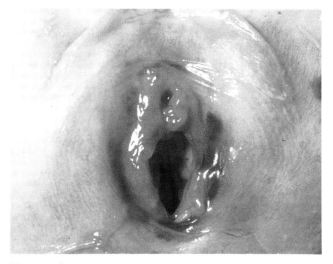

Fig. 123 Oedema and reddening of the vulva in a small child raped by an adult. There is copious bleeding from a lateral tear which had split the vaginal wall internally.

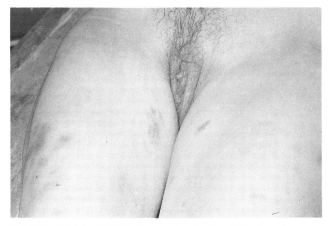

Fig. 124 Bruising of the thighs in a sexual assault. There are finger bruises on the inner side of the thighs, from attempts to force them apart, as well as on the lateral side, from forcible handling of the legs. Bruises and abrasions may also occur on the buttocks and shoulder-blades from contact with the ground.

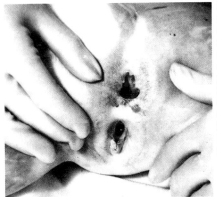

Fig. 125 Vulval and anal penetration in a sexual assault upon a small girl, who was manually strangled during the attack. The posterior margin of the vaginal orifice is torn and the anal sphincter is dilated, the edges being ripped in several places.

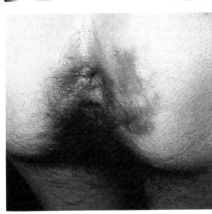

Fig. 126 The anus of a live victim of rape and buggery. The anus is lax but not injured, although semen was recovered on swabs. There is a prominent recent bruise on the adjacent buttock, due to manual manipulation to gain access.

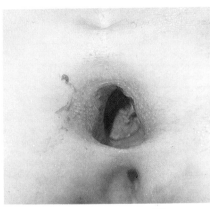

Fig. 127 The anus of a small girl who had recently been penetrated by an adult penis. There is dilatation of the orifice and some superficial tearing of the mucosal junction. In the dead, care must be taken not to over-interpret the normal laxity and even apparent dilatation of the anal ring.

Poisoning and alcohol

Most self-poisoning in advanced countries is now due to medicinal compounds, rather than corrosives or chemicals, but herbicides and insecticides, as well as irritant substances such as acids are still very common in more agricultural and developing lands. The spectrum of therapeutic drugs seen in suicides and accidental overdosage is vast and ever-increasing. Since the marked decline in barbiturate prescribing in Western countries, less toxic drugs are seen most often. Though the manufacturers may protest their relative safety, almost every drug has been used in over-dosage and it is can be very difficult or impossible to discover reliable data about expected toxic or fatal dosage or blood and tissue levels. There is great variation in the susceptibility of different people to the same amount of a drug - and the possibility of additive effects or multiple interaction has to be considered.

Often the post-mortem signs are unrewarding, as most therapeutic drugs even in great overdosage are not locally irritative or corrosive. Here, the diagnosis has to be entirely toxicologial and another problem then presents, the interpretation of blood, urine, liver and other tissue levels, especially when hard data are lacking with new drugs. Where death has been delayed, as in a prolonged period of coma before the victim was discovered, high blood levels may have declined to therapeutic or apparently non-lethal levels, due to elimination by excretion or detoxification processes. Sometimes liver levels or detection of the original drug or its breakdown products in the urine may give a truer picture of earlier high levels. '

Alcohol is a very important topic, both in the living and dead, in relation to behaviour, toxicity and the precipitation of violence.

Again, great variations exist between individuals and even the same individual at different times) in relation to rate of absorption, peak blood levels and most of all. Behaviour at any given blood level. It is dangerous to attempt to calculate the amount of drink that must have led to a given blood or urine level and conversely, to forecast the likely blood level from a knowledge of the amount of liquor imbibed. Only very approximate estimates, coupled with a warning of the potential inaccuracies, should be offered by way of an expert medical opinion.

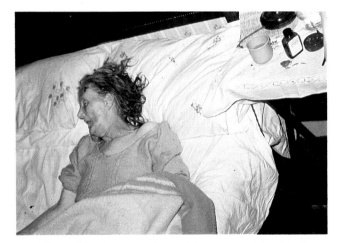

Fig. 128 A visit to the scene of a suspicious or unexplained death may assist the medical examiner. Here the dead woman has tablets on the bed-side table: although this is unremarkable, the nature of the drug may indicate what should be sought by the toxicology laboratory, if an overdose is suspected.

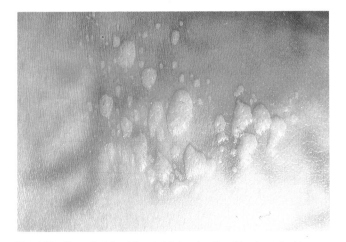

Fig. 129 So-called 'barbiturate blisters' on the skin of a patient in deep coma from phenobarbitone overdosage. Such blistering can be seen in any comatose patient, whether from poisoning (including carbon monoxide) or neurological causes. The blisters, which can be extensive, are usually in dependent parts such as legs, buttocks and shoulders.

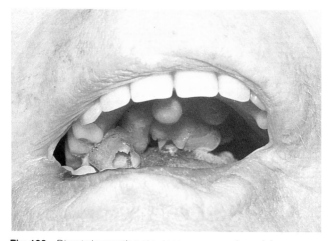

Fig. 130 Direct observation at autopsy may reveal suspicious or even obvious features. Here the mouth of a suicidal woman is filled with almost intact sodium amytal capsules. Capsules or tablets may be found in the clothing or bedding of dead persons. Sometimes dried vomit around the lips or on the clothing may reveal powder or coloured additives.

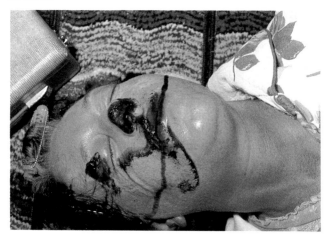

Fig. 131 Stomach contents around the nose and mouth from a barbiturate overdosage. The dark staining is caused by gastric bleeding from mucosal erosion due to the strongly alkaline sodium amytal.

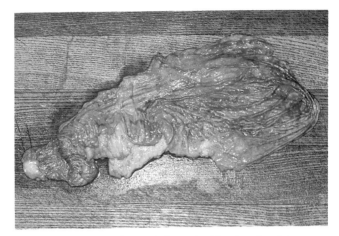

Fig. 132 Stomach and contents from a barbiturate poisoning, showing the turquoise coloration from the capsule dye used in sodium amytal preparations. At autopsy, intact or partially dissolved capsules and tablets should be carefully retained for examination, as well as powder, sludge and liquid required for chemical analysis.

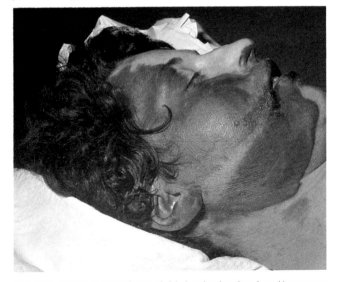

Fig. 133 Facial staining from suicide lysol poisoning. Lysol is a soapy compound of phenol and is caustic to skin. This damage is due to regurgitation, the direction of flow indicating that the victim was lying down.

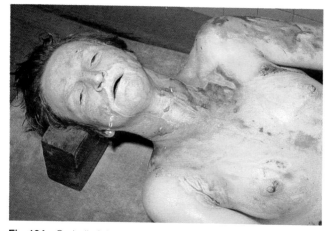

Fig. 134 Carbolic (phenol) poisoning. The skin damage here is due to spillage, rather than vomiting, as it has occurred whilst the victim was standing up.

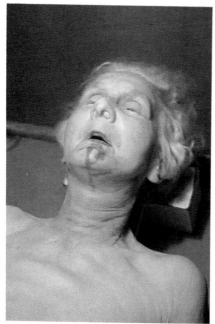

Fig. 135 Suicide from hydrochloric acid. The external signs are relatively slight in this particular case, as the acid was not very concentrated. However, oesophageal and gastric damage was eventually fatal. Corrosive poisons such as these have been largely replaced in advanced countries by easily obtainable medicinal drugs, which rarely leave visible signs, their detection being a task for the laboratory.

ABSORBTION

Hastened by:-
Empty stomach
20% alcohol
Gasto-enterostomy

Retarded by:-
Full stomach
Weak or very
strong alcohol
Fatty meal

(Partial gastrectomy)

BLOOD LEVEL

30 mg/100 ml

Empty stomach

Approximate
blood response
to 1 pint beer
(very variable)

With meal

0   1   2   3

Hours

ELIMINATION

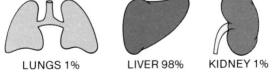

LUNGS 1%   LIVER 98%   KIDNEY 1%

Blood level falls at approximately
15 mg/100 ml per hour
(range 12–20) after drinking ceases.

Fig. 136 Alcohol: Diagrammatic summary of factors affecting the
rate of absorption, the blood levels and rate of elimination. It must
always be appreciated that no *accurate* estimate of the blood level can
be made from a knowledge of the amount of drink consumed nor the
converse.

Index

Entries in **bold** refer to Fig. numbers